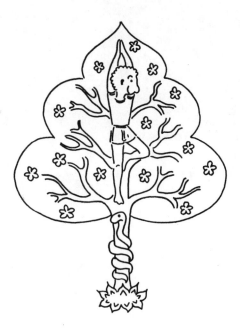

THE
HATHA YOGA
WORKBOOK

Based on
HATHA YOGA: THE HIDDEN LANGUAGE
by Swami Sivananda Radha

D1605223

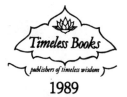

Timeless Books
publishers of timeless wisdom
1989

Acknowledgment is given to Mary Armstrong for her insightful suggestion to produce this workbook based on *Hatha Yoga: The Hidden Language.*

Illustrations by Linda Pelton
Book design by Cynthia Poole
Front cover illustrations by Linda Pelton

©1989 by Swami Sivananda Radha

ISBN 0-931454-15-8

Hidden Language Hatha Yoga™

The Hidden Language approach to Hatha Yoga can only be taught by those certified in this technique through the Yasodhara Ashram or its affiliated centers. Information is available from Yasodhara Ashram, Box 9, Kootenay Bay, B.C. V0B 1X0

Published by

Timeless Books

Box 160
Porthill, ID 83853

ABOUT THIS JOURNAL

Why would anyone want or need a journal for Hatha Yoga? If Hatha Yoga were just physical exercise there would be little need to write anything down except the "how-to's." But Hatha is much more than that, as Swami Sivananda Radha has shown in *Hatha Yoga: The Hidden Language,* the companion text to this journal. Her approach to Hatha Yoga very quickly brings you to the deeper meanings of the asanas—the psychological and spiritual meanings hidden within each posture.

Using her method, you discover the deeper meanings by asking yourself a question related to the posture you are doing: for example, while doing *paschimottanasana,* the Sitting Forward Bend, you may ask yourself, What does it mean to bend forward? Let the question open within you, not "trying" to come up with an answer. Use this journal to write down whatever comes to you. Sometimes nothing will come. Sometimes an image, a word, a feeling, or a complete insight will appear. Let the question enter your daily life for the next week and see what else emerges. Questions have been suggested (either on their own or in conjunction with the cartoon characters) for you to try with each asana. Swami Sivananda Radha's book, *Hatha Yoga: The Hidden Language* presents many more questions as well as a wealth of insights into the symbolism of the postures.

So—a journal for doing Hatha Yoga. But a *cartoon* journal? Is Hatha Yoga funny? I have cartooned since I was about four years old, but I give credit to Swami Radha for helping me see why cartooning and why humor, are so important. It is easy to take spiritual life so very seriously. To take myself so very seriously. Plymouth Rock. John Calvin. Sin and Purgatory. Humor puts my problems into perspective and provides the relaxation that is so essential if change is to occur. I can't surrender to and be receptive to the wisdom within if I don't relax. Surrender *is* relaxation.

Do animals laugh? Snakes? Ants? Zebras? I suspect no. I suspect that only humans laugh because only humans have egos, and so experience the kinds of stresses and strains that make laughter a necessity. One of those stresses is over-conscientious scrupulosity—spiritual fastidiousness. We really need a poke in the ribs from time to time to get us out of that one.

Someone once gave me the prescription of "a belly laugh a day." Keeps the over-conscientious scrupulosity away.

Not a bad idea.

Yours truly, in good humor,

Linda Pelton

Linda Pelton
Illustrator

THE ASANAS (in sequence)

STRUCTURES

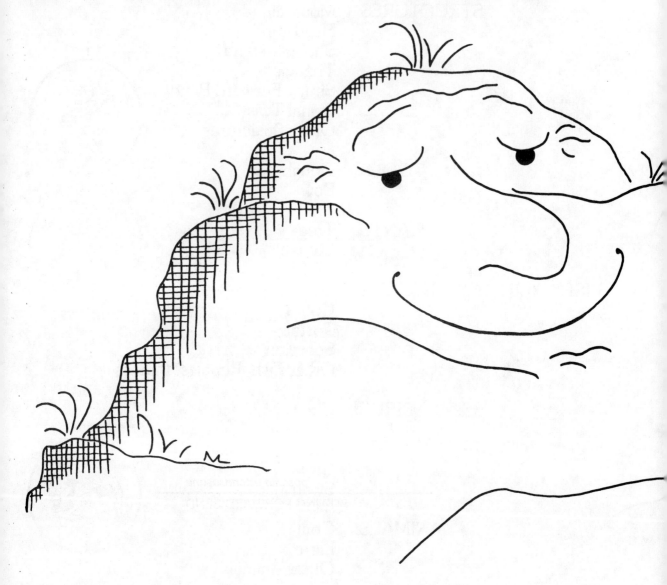

tadasana
MOUNTAIN

salamba shirshasana
HEADSTAND

salamba sarvangasana
SHOULDERSTAND

utthita trikonasana
TRIANGLE

paschimottanasasana
SITTING FORWARD BEND

ardha matsyendrasana
SPINAL TWIST

tadasana
MOUNTAIN

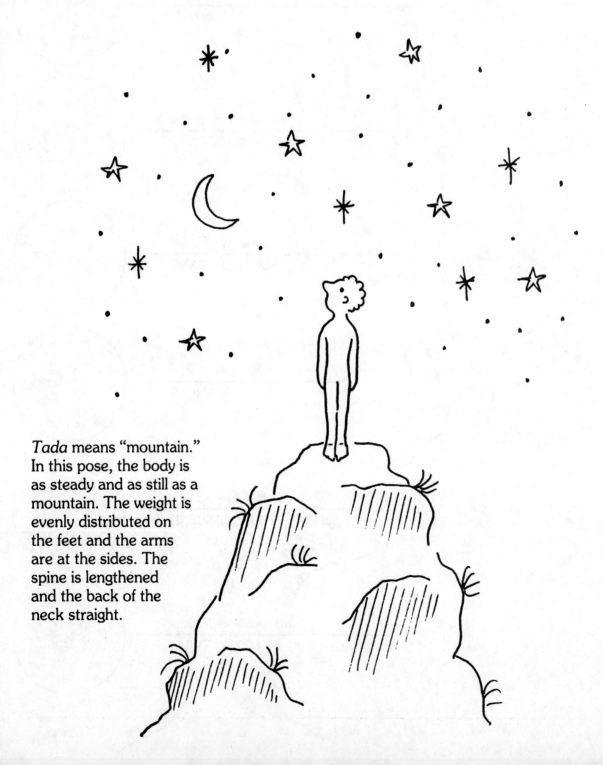

Tada means "mountain." In this pose, the body is as steady and as still as a mountain. The weight is evenly distributed on the feet and the arms are at the sides. The spine is lengthened and the back of the neck straight.

MY REFLECTIONS ON MOUNTAIN:

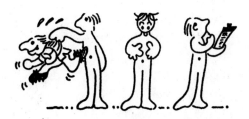

Standing still: not running somewhere
Standing still: looking without, within
Standing still: taking stock

tadasana

MOUNTAIN

Where do I stand on important principles, ideals, ethics, decisions, beliefs, convictions?

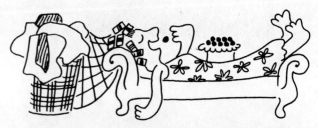

It can become quite evident that the mind is not willing,
or "in the mood," to concentrate.

tadasana

MOUNTAIN

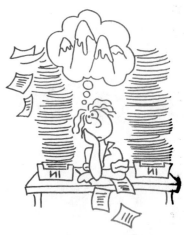

It is during the time of reflection
that the student can use the
symbolic meaning of the postures
and their names to deal with
irritations and problems.

tadasana

MOUNTAIN

Who stands: a person? an actor? a shell?

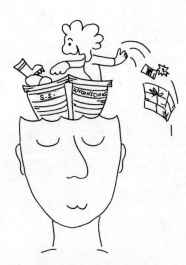

The unconscious will use this quiet, relaxed opportunity to throw off as much "ballast" as possible.

tadasana

MOUNTAIN

What does a mountain mean to me?

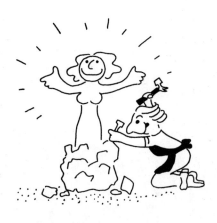

Positive personal experience through
one's own efforts, and under the
hammer of repetition, will slowly
chip away undesirable characteristics.

tadasana

MOUNTAIN

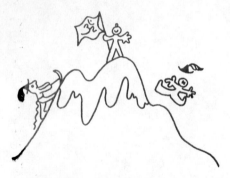

Ascending, descending, being on top

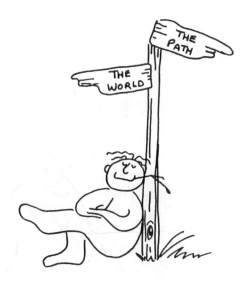

Being lukewarm you are neither
in the world nor on the "Path."

tadasana

MOUNTAIN

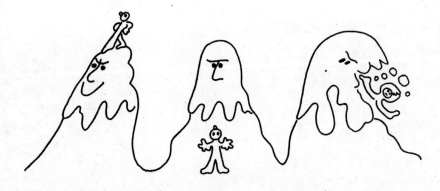

Power . . . obstacles . . . avalanches

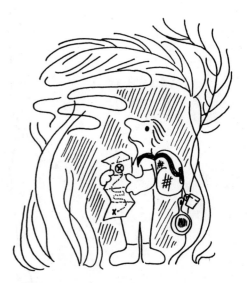

Those practicing Yoga must be encouraged to discover unknown territory by themselves.

tadasana

MOUNTAIN

salamba shirshasana
HEADSTAND

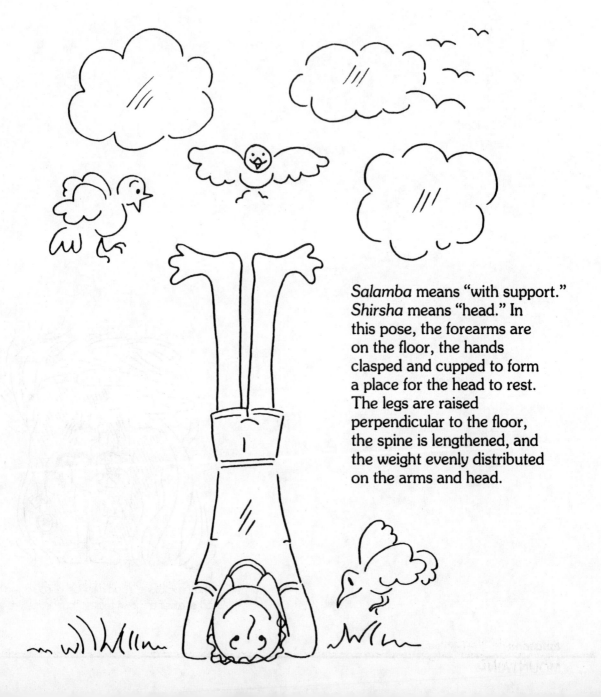

Salamba means "with support."
Shirsha means "head." In
this pose, the forearms are
on the floor, the hands
clasped and cupped to form
a place for the head to rest.
The legs are raised
perpendicular to the floor,
the spine is lengthened, and
the weight evenly distributed
on the arms and head.

MY REFLECTIONS ON HEADSTAND:

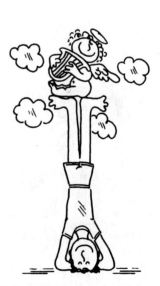

In the headstand, that which has
been rooted in the earth becomes rooted in heaven.

salamba shirshasana

HEADSTAND

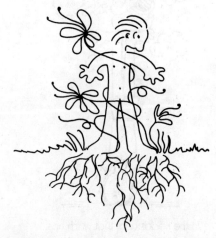

What does it mean to be "earth-bound"?

salamba shirshasana

HEADSTAND

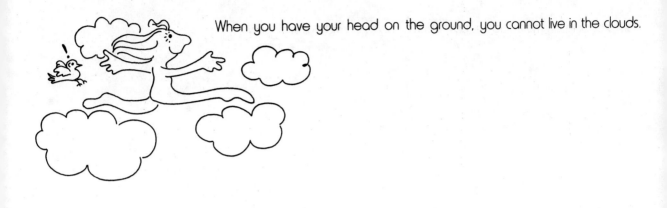

When you have your head on the ground, you cannot live in the clouds.

salamba shirshasana

HEADSTAND

I am standing on my head — how do my strong convictions look now?

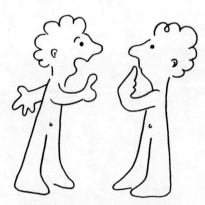

If you meet with strong opposition
to your convictions, become your own
opponent and take the other side
of the argument.

salamba shirshasana

HEADSTAND

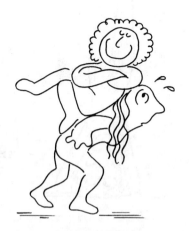

It is not your task to carry
the weight of, or the responsibility
for, anyone else.

salamba shirshasana

HEADSTAND

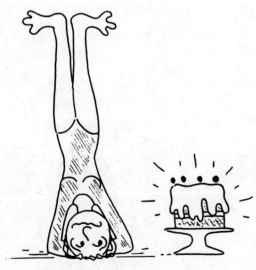

There are many movements
— to fulfill ambitions and gratify desires —
that cannot be made when you are
standing on your head.

salamba shirshasana

HEADSTAND

What would happen if my life was turned upside down?

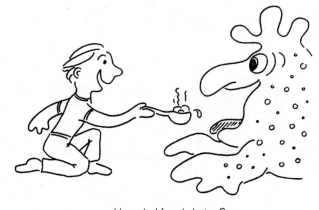

How do I feed desires?

salamba shirshasana

HEADSTAND

salamba sarvangasana
SHOULDERSTAND

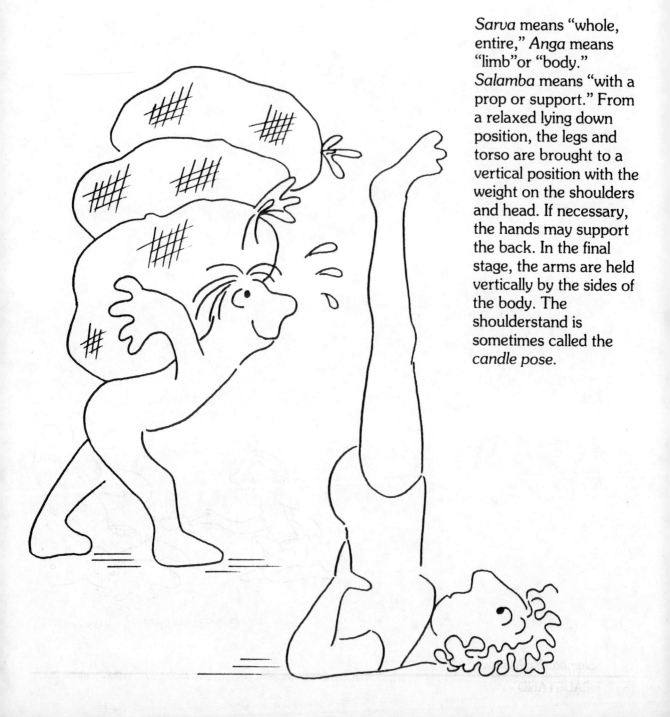

Sarva means "whole, entire," *Anga* means "limb" or "body." *Salamba* means "with a prop or support." From a relaxed lying down position, the legs and torso are brought to a vertical position with the weight on the shoulders and head. If necessary, the hands may support the back. In the final stage, the arms are held vertically by the sides of the body. The shoulderstand is sometimes called the *candle pose.*

MY REFLECTIONS ON SHOULDERSTAND:

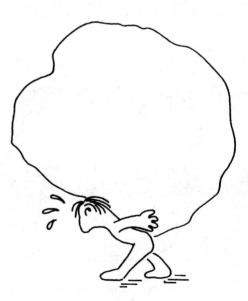

What burdens can I put down?

salamba sarvangasana

SHOULDERSTAND

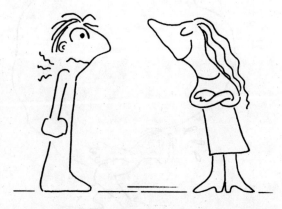

Pains in the neck are either self-created
or come from others who will not bend to our will.

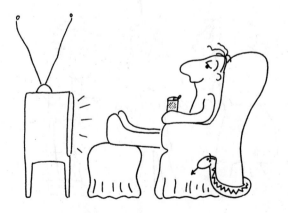

When everything is comfortable and pleasant,
human beings become complacent.

salamba sarvangasana

SHOULDERSTAND

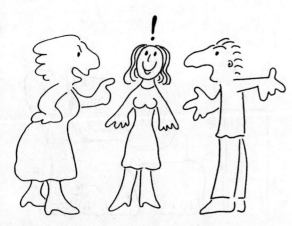

Awareness is not increased one iota
unless we are put under pressure.

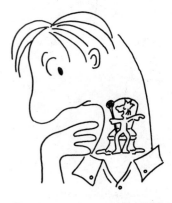

The throat is the seat of self-will.

salamba sarvangasana

SHOULDERSTAND

What burdens are no longer mine?

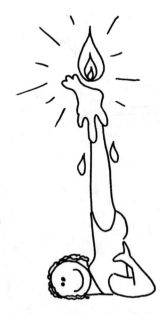

The *candle pose:* I can help to "lighten" myself.

salamba sarvangasana

SHOULDERSTAND

TRIANGLE

Utthita means "extended," *tri* means "three," and *kona* is "an angle." This is the extended triangle, which is done first to one side and then to the other. The legs spread apart and the body stretches to the left, moving from the pelvis and extending over the left leg. Both arms are perpendicular to the floor, the left hand on the floor, or grasping the outer ankle of the left foot, and the right hand reaching up straight. The spine is straight, the chest is open, the body facing to the front.

MY REFLECTIONS ON TRIANGLE:

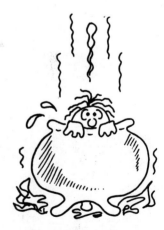

Originally, a tripod was
a caldron with three legs,
used for cooking food over fire.

utthita trikonasana

TRIANGLE

How much can I resist pressure?

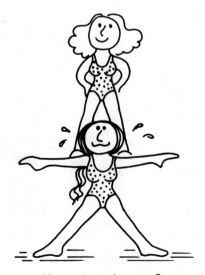

How much can I support?

utthita trikonasana

TRIANGLE

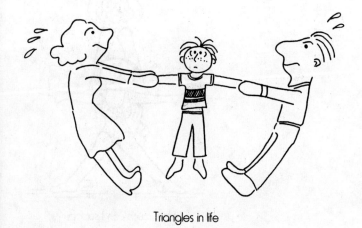

Triangles in life

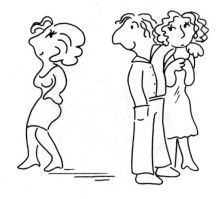

Triangles in life

utthita trikonasana

TRIANGLE

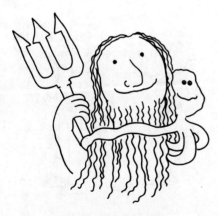

Neptune and his trident

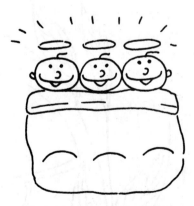

In times past, the birth of triplets
was taken as a special blessing of the deity.

utthita trikonasana

TRIANGLE

paschimottanasana

SITTING FORWARD BEND

Paschima means "the west." This pose stretches the western part of the body, which is the entire back from the head to the heels. From a sitting position with the legs extended straight out, the upper body stretches up from the pelvis, arms over the head. The upper body bends forward, the hands reaching toward the feet. Relaxing into the pose creates a sense of releasing into a place of surrender and humility.

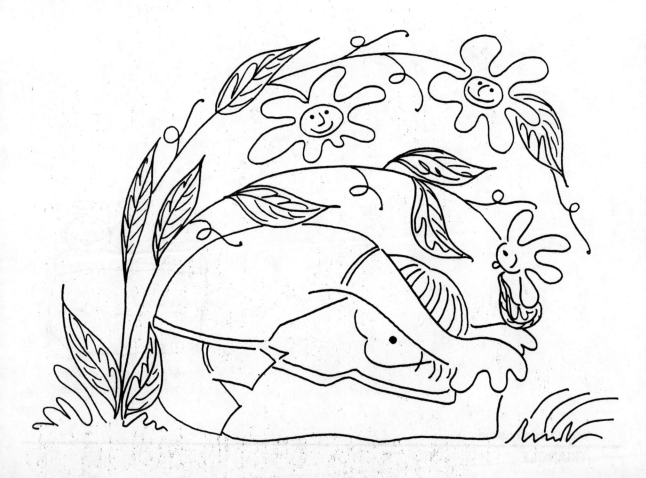

MY REFLECTIONS ON SITTING FORWARD BEND:

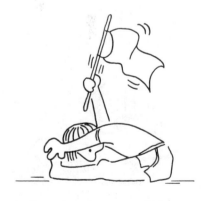

Surrender is the important lesson
that this asana teaches.

paschimottanasana

SITTING FORWARD BEND

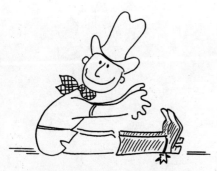

The Sanskrit word *Paschimottanasana*
means "intense stretch to the west."

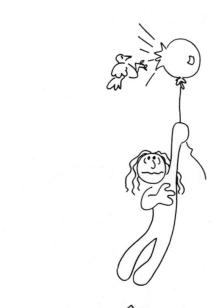

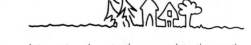

It is coming down to the ground, to the earth,
that makes not for the ending of life, but for a beginning.

paschimottanasana

SITTING FORWARD BEND

Can the separation of good and bad, like white and black, really be established?

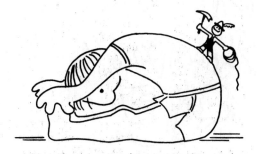

Before one can fold with a straight spine, there is often a big hump, an obstacle, that one has to get over.

paschimottanasana

SITTING FORWARD BEND

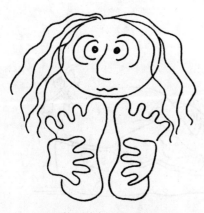

In this pose, one must accept
the insecurity of limited vision.

paschimottanasana

SITTING FORWARD BEND

Can there really be a broken circuit of energy, or a divided circle?

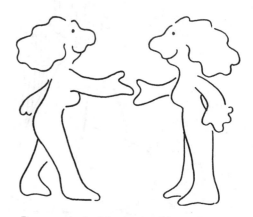

The need to trust the innate divine nature

paschimottanasana

SITTING FORWARD BEND

ardha matsyendrasana

SPINAL TWIST

Ardha means "half." *Matsyendra* was a sage who spread the teachings of Yoga. In this pose, the left leg is on the floor and bent so that the foot is on the outside of the right buttock. The right leg is bent and upright with the foot on the outside of the left thigh. The body twists to the right with the left arm passed around the bent knee of the right leg, the hands clasped behind the back. The head turns to the right to look behind. The pose is repeated on the other side.

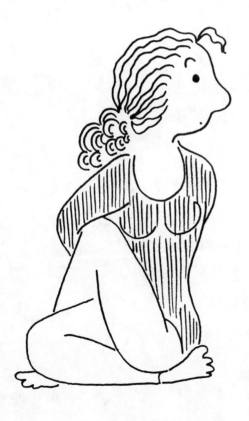

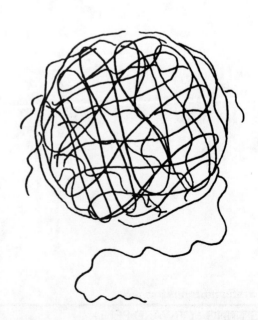

MY REFLECTIONS ON SPINAL TWIST:

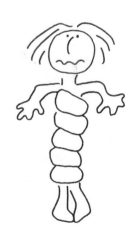

If the body is tied
in a knot, so are
the mind and the emotions.

ardha matsyendrasana

TWIST

Can I go back to the basic event, before there was any bending and twisting? To unravel a problem you can go through each movement in the mind as you do in the asana.

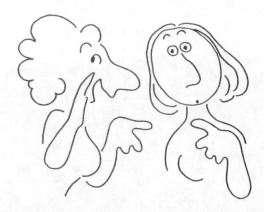

There is little that does not get twisted to some degree — such as stories that we hear and retell.

ardha matsyendrasana

TWIST

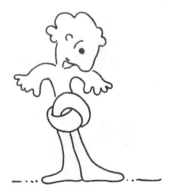

For every mental problem or knot,
there is a corresponding
knot in the body,
and vice versa.

ardha matsyendrasana

TWIST

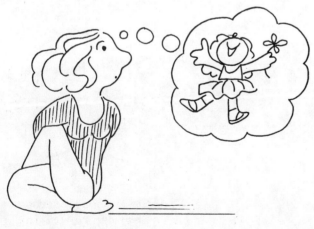

Looking back . . .

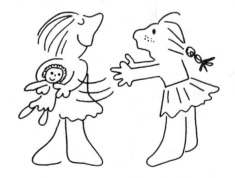

Sometimes the mind is so flexible
that it can twist from "thine" to "mine"
and "mine" to "thine."

ardha matsyendrasana

TWIST

You want the body to be flexible and supple; do you want your mind also to be flexible and supple?

ardha matsyendrasana

TWIST

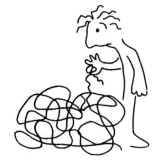

What has been twisted can also be untwisted.

ardha matsyendrasana

TWIST

MY REFLECTIONS ON OTHER STRUCTURES:

additional
STRUCTURES

additional
STRUCTURES

TOOLS

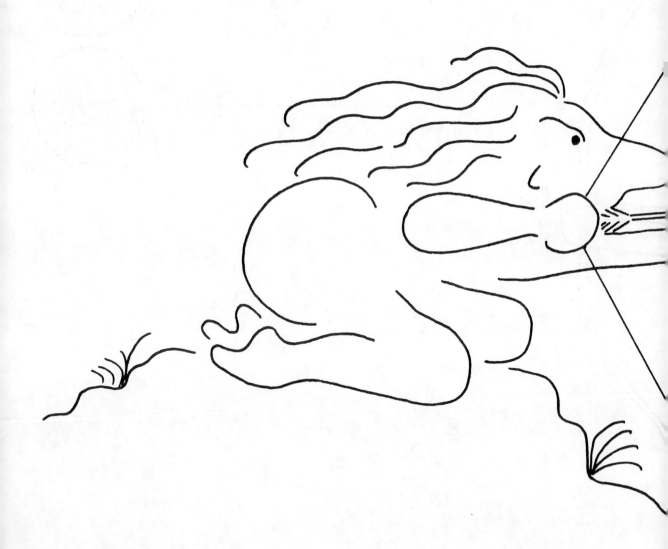

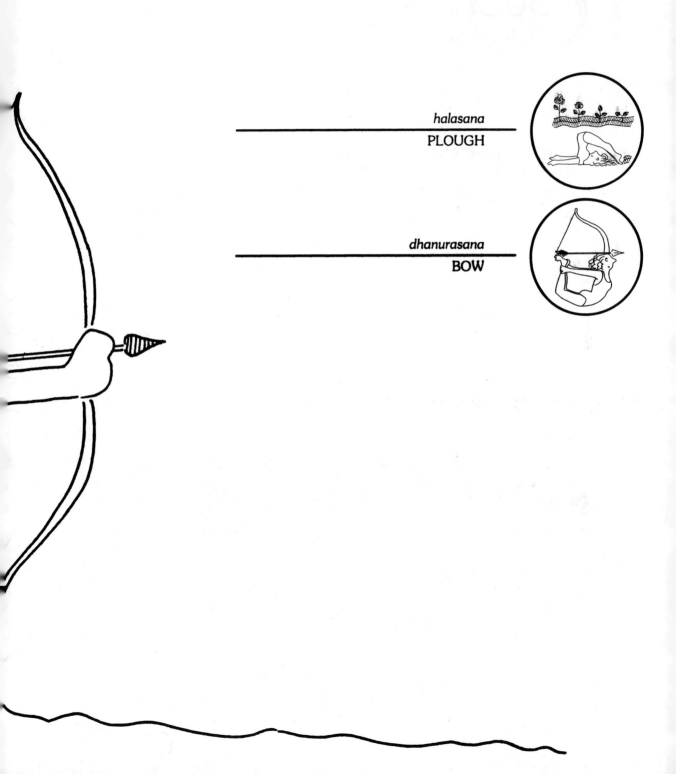

halasana
PLOUGH

dhanurasana
BOW

halasana

PLOUGH

Hala means "plough." From a relaxed position lying down with the arms at the sides, the feet are brought over the head toward the ground. The arms and feet remain relaxed. The position suggests a plough.

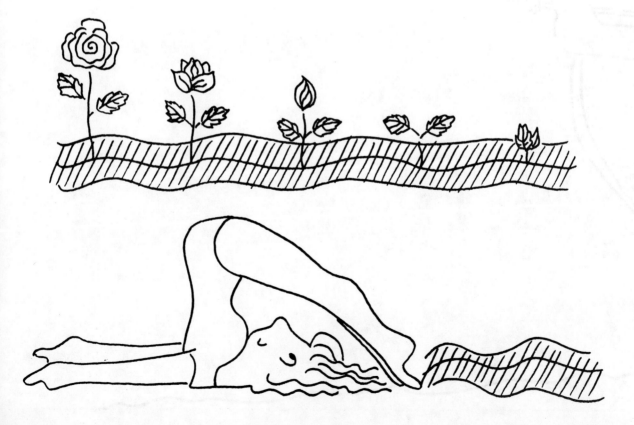

MY REFLECTIONS ON PLOUGH:

What am I ploughing through in my life?

halasana

PLOUGH

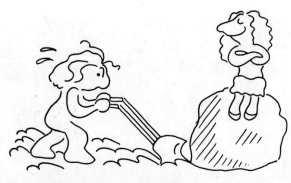

"What are the hard lumps I must break up?"

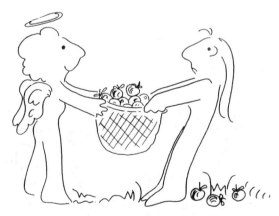

The *Bhagavad Gita* tells us that we
should renounce the fruits of our labor,
and dedicate them to the Divine.

halasana

Is the security in my life constricting me?

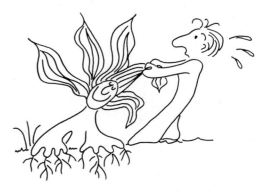

Weeds — concepts that have, like crabgrass, grown deep — are hard to remove.

halasana

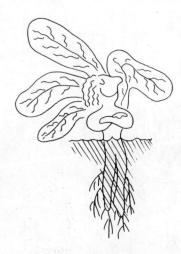

Discrimination is needed to
distinguish good healthy thoughts
from the weeds of self-importance.

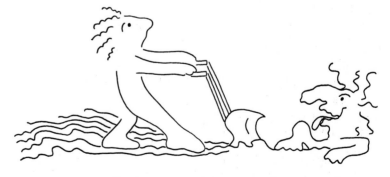

Ploughing turns up the unexpected.

halasana

PLOUGH

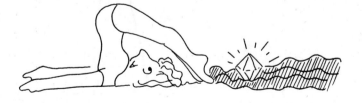

The plough may reveal hidden treasure.

halasana

PLOUGH

dhanurasana

BOW

Dhanu means "bow." The pose starts from a downward-facing position. The hands are brought back to grasp the ankles. As the legs, chest, and head lift up, the movement suggests the tensing of a bow, bent and aimed at the target.

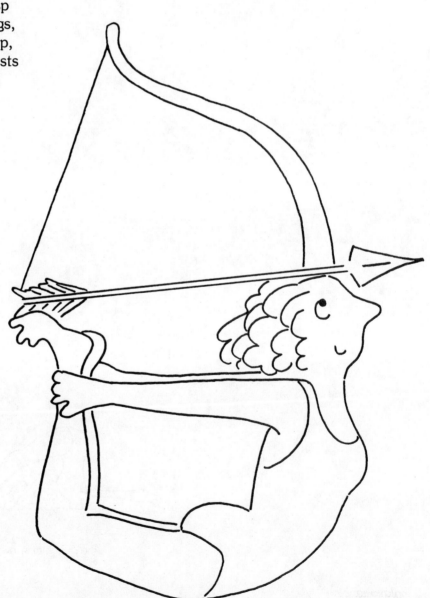

MY REFLECTIONS ON BOW:

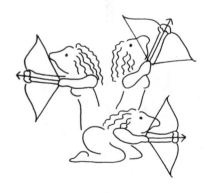

What are you aiming for?

Is the main target well-defined, clear?

dhanurasana

BOW

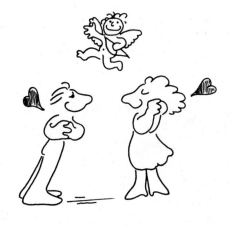

Cupid's bow

dhanurasana

BOW

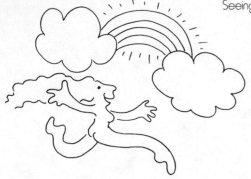

Seeing a rainbow usually evokes a feeling of hope and optimism.

dhanurasana

BOW

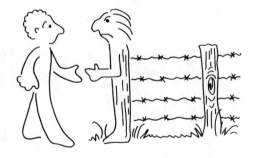

To be in accord with others, you must bend equally
from end to end, and not resist stiffly like a post.

dhanurasana

BOW

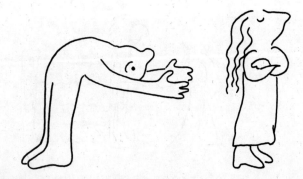

We will bend over backwards for the sake of acceptance from others.

dhanurasana

BOW

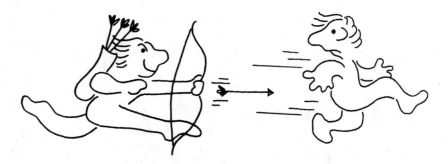

To hit the spiritual goal, you must aim at yourself.

dhanurasana

BOW

PLANTS

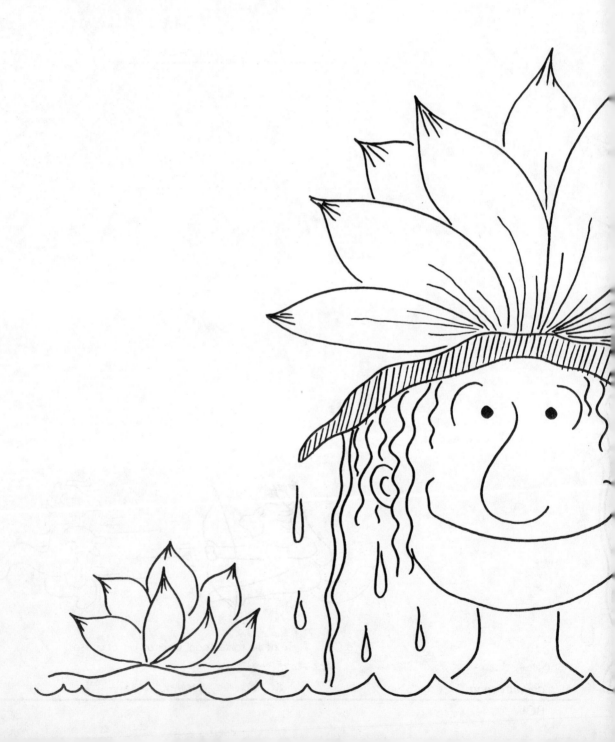

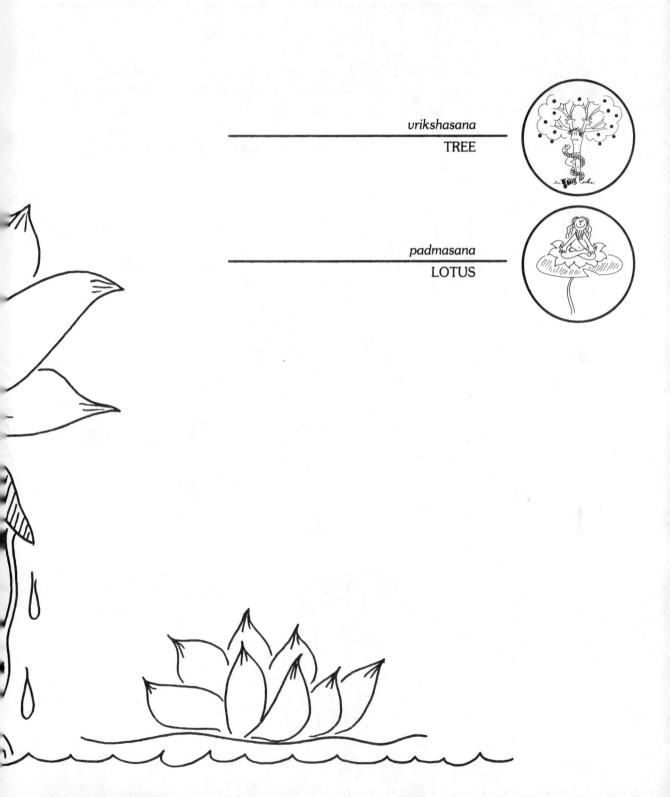

vrikshasana
TREE

padmasana
LOTUS

vrikshasana

TREE

Vriksha means "tree." In this posture, a steady, rooted stance is created by bringing one foot against the inner thigh of the other, standing, leg. The knee of the raised leg is out to the side and the pelvis opened. The arms are raised from the namaste position at the chest and are stretched up over the head, just as the limbs of a tree lift to the sunlight. The pose is repeated on the opposite side.

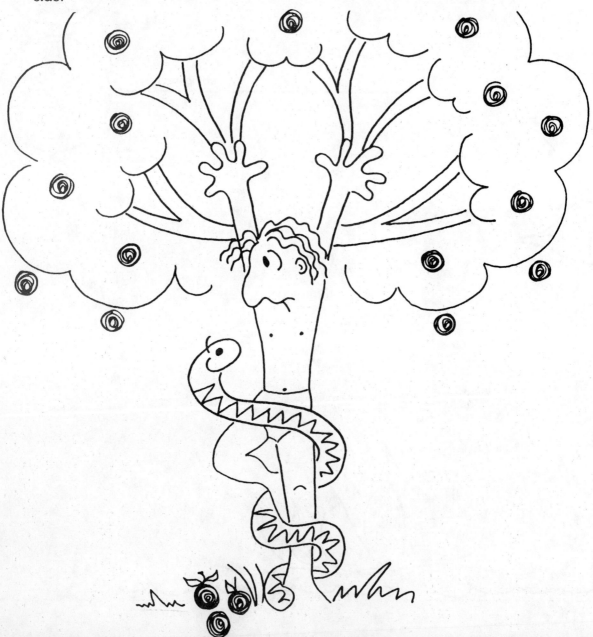

MY REFLECTIONS ON TREE:

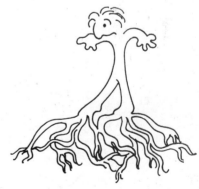

Where have my roots spread?
Where do they get their nourishment?
Which are mine and which belong to someone else?

vrikshasana

TREE

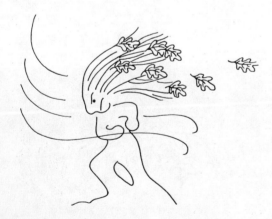

The oak must let go of too much strength,
    too much resistance . . .

vrikshasana

TREE

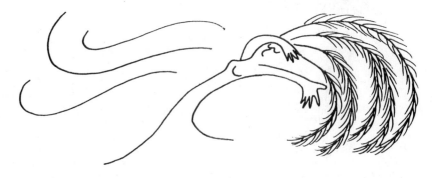

. . . The willow must not allow itself to be beaten to the ground by the whims of destiny.

vrikshasana

TREE

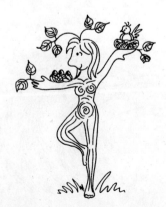

Wherever the tree is, it must share.

vrikshasana

TREE

What competes with my roots for nourishment?

vrikshasana

TREE

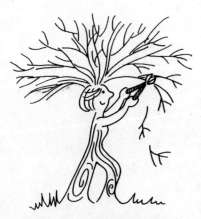

The aspirant must prune branches
that are not productive,
and cut away side growth.

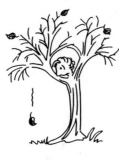

Drying up

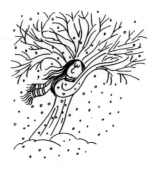

Dormancy

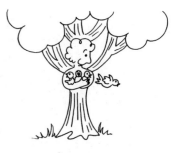

Protective

vrikshasana

TREE

padmasana
LOTUS

Padma means "lotus." In
this posture the legs are
crossed, the feet rest-
ing on the thighs with
the soles facing up.
The spine is erect,
the hands either
placed on the
knees, palms
up, or resting
in the lap.

MY REFLECTIONS ON LOTUS:

What prevents me from achieving the Royal Posture?

padmasana

LOTUS

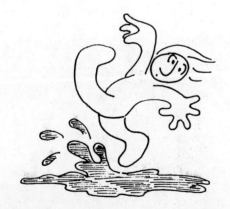

The waters of selfishness are muddy and slippery.

padmasana

LOTUS

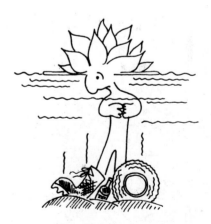

The lotus does not grow in crystal clear streams,
but in the collected debris that has sunk to the bottom of the lake.

padmasana

LOTUS

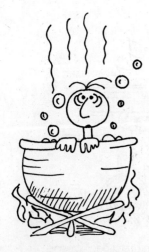

Getting into hot water

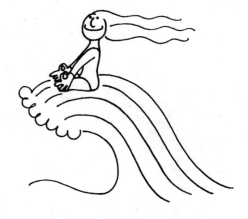

Riding the crest of the wave

padmasana

LOTUS

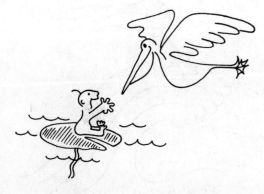

In children's stories, the stork picks up babies
from the leaf of the lotus or water lily.

padmasana

LOTUS

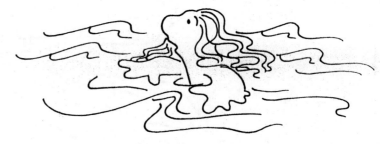

It is only through the pursuit of Divine Wisdom
that one can, like the lotus flower, keep one's head above
the surface of the turbulent waters of life.

padmasana

LOTUS

FISH, REPTILES, INSECTS

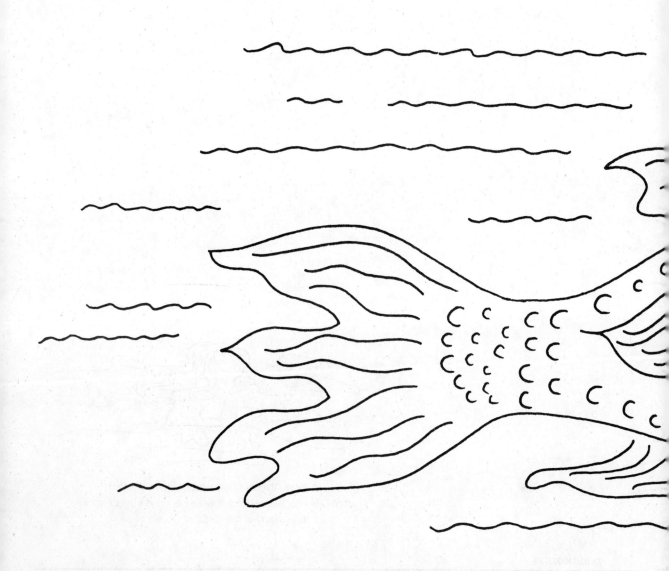

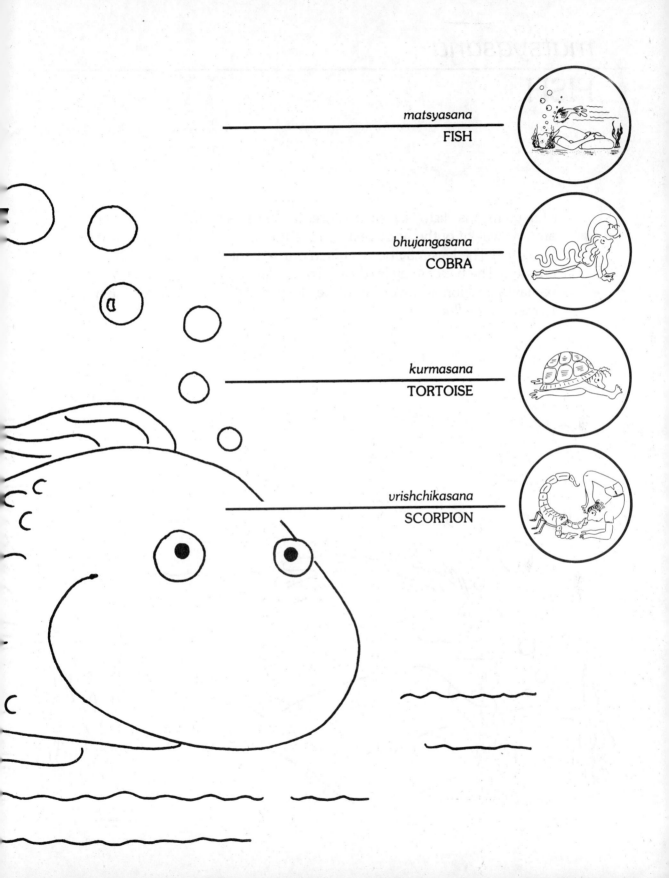

matsyasana
FISH

bhujangasana
COBRA

kurmasana
TORTOISE

vrishchikasana
SCORPION

matsyasana

FISH

Matsya means "fish." In this posture, the chest is open, the spine arched, and the weight of the body rests on the top of the head and the base of the spine. The legs may be stretched out or bent at the knees and crossed. The hands may hold the crossed feet, or be placed in the namaste position at the chest, or be clasped at the elbows over the head to rest on the floor.

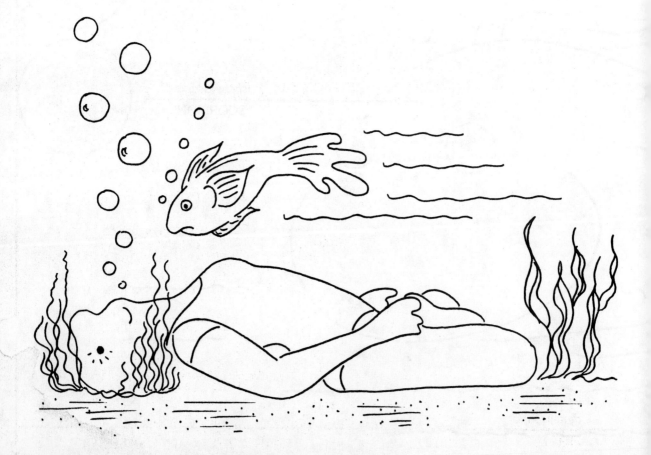

MY REFLECTIONS ON FISH:

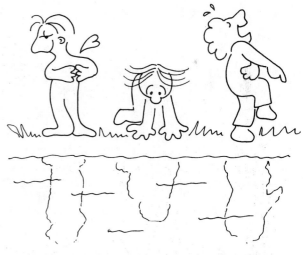

Humans everywhere have been fascinated with the reflections of themselves on the quiet surface of water.

matsyasana

FISH

What am I lifting up — my lungs, my heart? Why that strain on my throat, my neck?

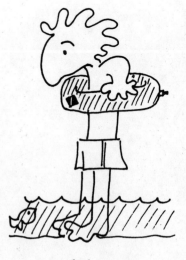

Can't swim

matsyasana

FISH

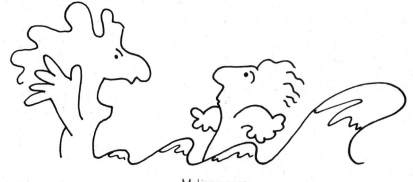

Making waves

How much can anybody see when flooded with emotions?

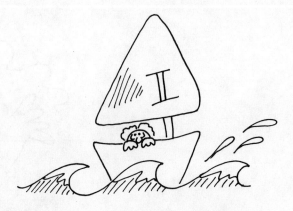

Fear of water

matsyasana

FISH

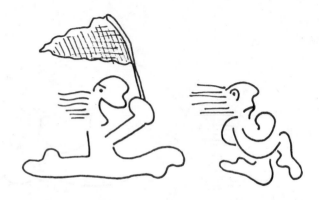

Watching out for the net so as not to be caught

matsyasana

FISH

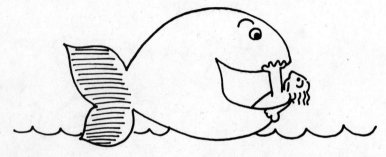

Jonah in the belly of the fish

matsyasana

FISH

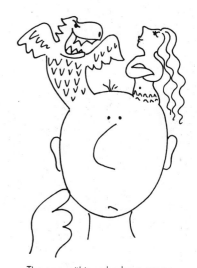

The sea within us harbors many
creatures of our imagination — frightening
monsters and beautiful mermaids.

matsyasana

FISH

bhujangasana

COBRA

Bhujanga means "serpent." The pose starts from a downward-facing position with the palms of the hands flat on the floor below the shoulders. The spine is lengthened and the buttocks firmed as the head and chest are slowly lifted. The elbows stay close to the body and the eyes look up. The return to the original position is made slowly.

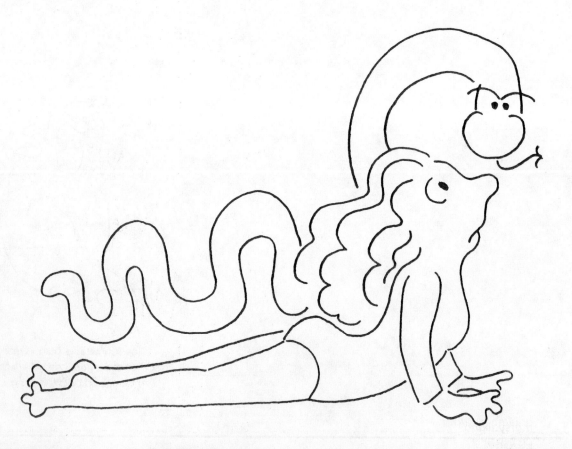

MY REFLECTIONS ON COBRA:

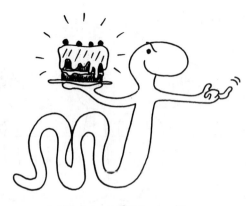

In the Judaeo-Christian tradition,
the snake is temptation.

bhujangasana

COBRA

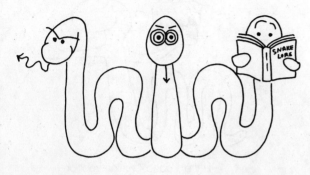

The snake: demonic . . . magnetic . . . wise . . .

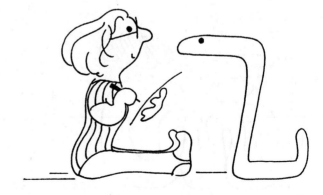

What else does a snake mean to me? What can I learn from it?

bhujangasana

COBRA

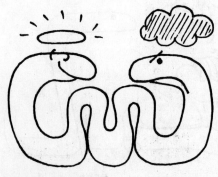

The two-headed serpent is good and evil.

bhujangasana

COBRA

How can I shed my old skin?

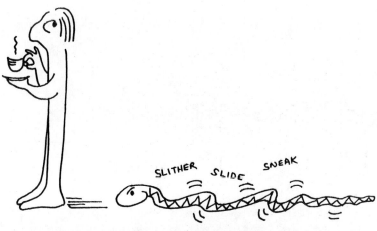

SLITHER SLIDE SNEAK

Snakes move almost noiselessly: evil approaches in the same way.

bhujangasana

COBRA

What are the poisons of my mind? Can I watch at all times?

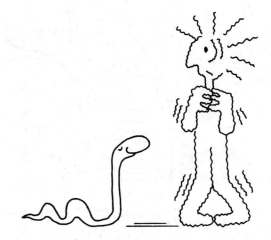

There are very few people who are not afraid of snakes.

bhujangasana

COBRA

kurmasana

TORTOISE

Kurma means "tortoise," and the final stage of the pose resembles a tortoise withdrawn into its shell. In the first stage, the legs are over the arms which are outstretched on either side of the body, chest and shoulders on the floor. In the next stage, the hands are brought behind the body palms up. In the final stage, Supta Kurmasana, the feet are crossed, the arms behind the back with the hands clasped, the forehead on the floor.

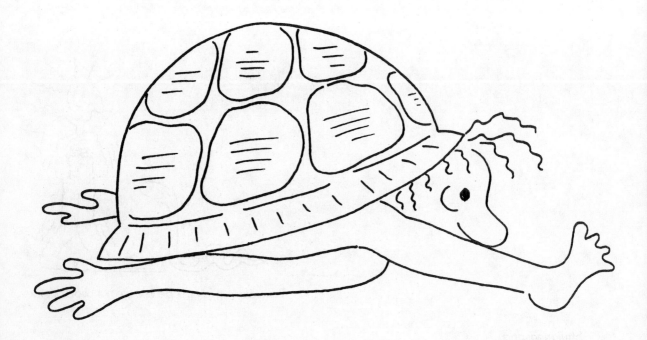

MY REFLECTIONS ON TORTOISE:

What is your shell made of? . . .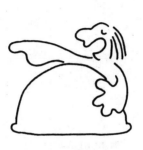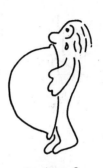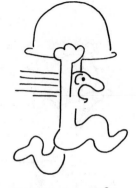

sarcasm? . . .　　　touchiness? . . .　　　tendency to panic? . . .

kurmasana

TORTOISE

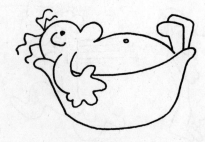

Vulnerable

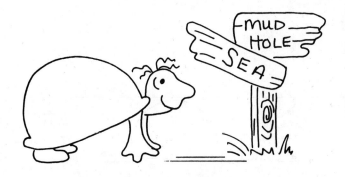

The belief is that the tortoise never gets lost.

kurmasana

TORTOISE

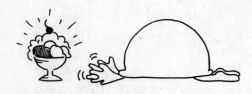

Avoiding seeing temptations

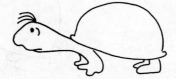

Sticking one's neck out

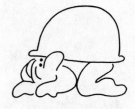

Self-protecting

kurmasana

TORTOISE

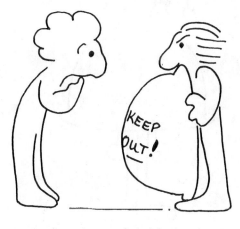

Intensifying one's shell for the
purpose of keeping people from
coming too close is not helpful.

kurmasana

TORTOISE

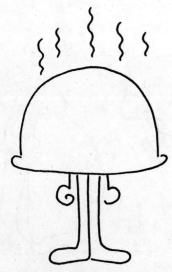

Retreating into the shell can help
the hot-tempered person become
calm and composed.

kurmasana

TORTOISE

Will I ever find that inner place of rest?

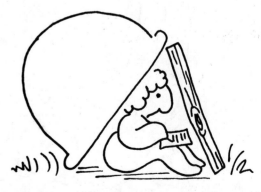

Retreating to get thoughts and emotions under control

kurmasana

TORTOISE

vrishchikasana

SCORPION

Vrishchika means "scorpion," the creature this pose resembles. With the forearms resting on the floor, the legs are raised up, and the head and chest lifted. The legs are bent at the knees, and the feet lowered slowly behind the back until they rest on the crown of the head.

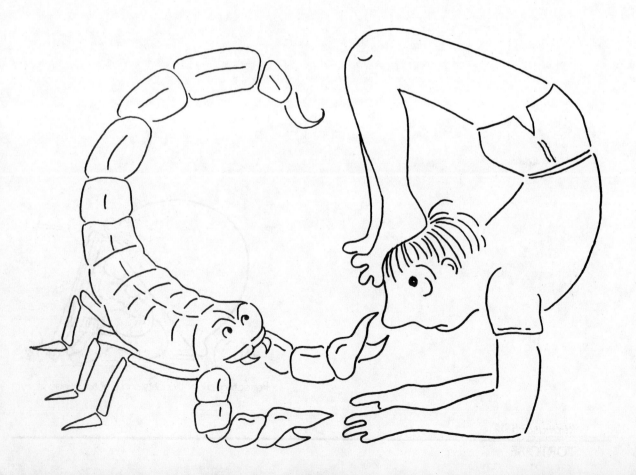

MY REFLECTIONS ON SCORPION:

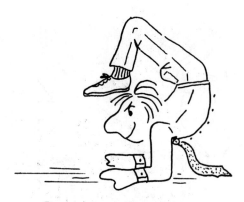

The scorpion is a dangerous creature,
easily excited, attacking
without proper discrimination.

vrishchikasana

SCORPION

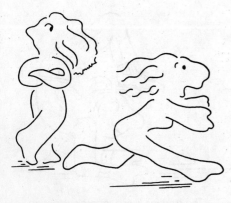

Do I respond to the needs of people with
scorpion-like quickness, or do I speculate
whether the individual is worth my time?

Would I like to have the sensitivity to respond with a scorpion-like quickness to even an unspoken need?

vrishchikasana
SCORPION

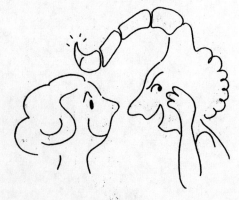

The sting

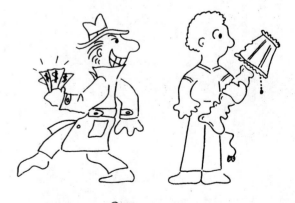

Getting stung

vrishchikasana
SCORPION

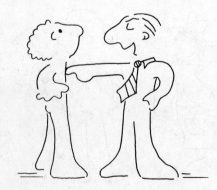

Am I stinging people to hurt them?

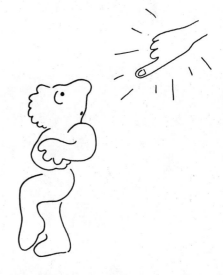

Allow the Divine Forces to sting your self-glorification.

vrishchikasana

SCORPION

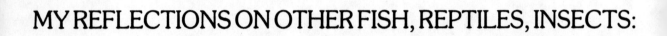

MY REFLECTIONS ON OTHER FISH, REPTILES, INSECTS:

additional
FISH, REPTILES, INSECTS

BIRDS

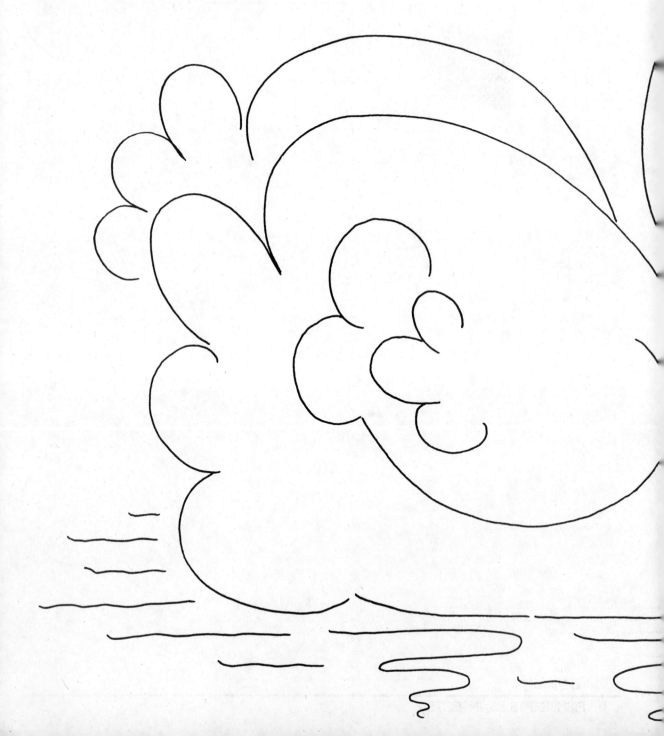

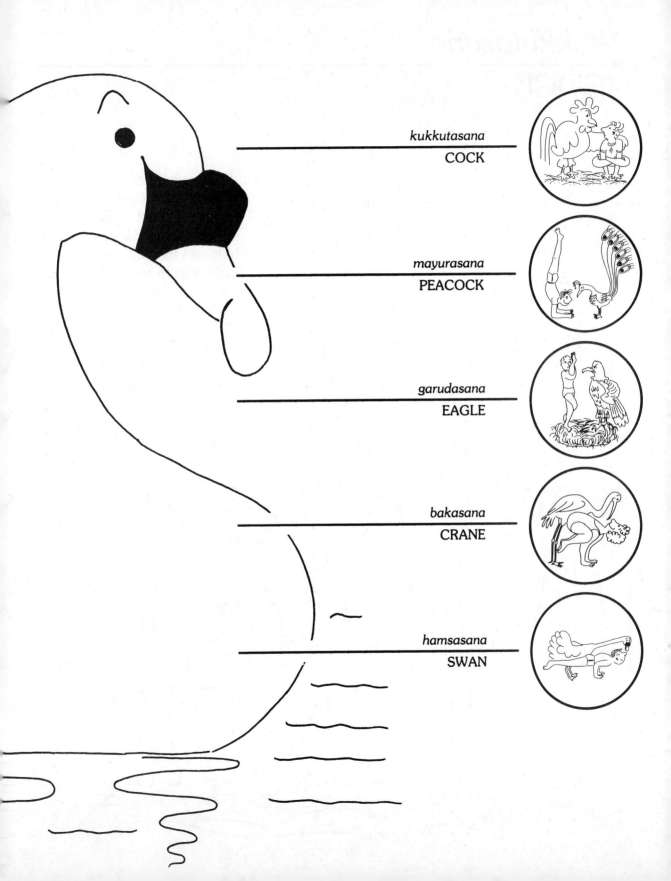

kukkutasana
COCK

mayurasana
PEACOCK

garudasana
EAGLE

bakasana
CRANE

hamsasana
SWAN

kukkutasana

COCK

Kukkuta means "cock." With the legs crossed in Padmasana, the hands and arms are placed between the calf and thigh of each leg, and the body is raised off the floor in a position that resembles a cock. The pose is repeated with the legs crossed in the opposite way.

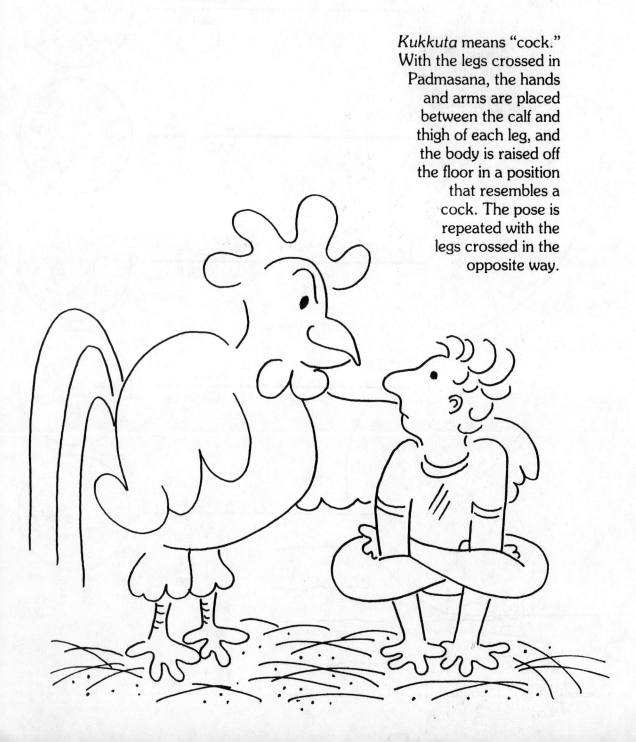

MY REFLECTIONS ON COCK:

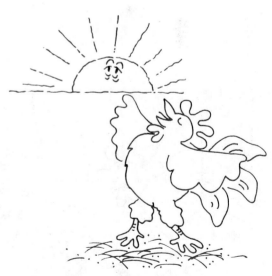

The Chinese believe that it is the cock's
well-accepted duty to awaken the glorious sun.

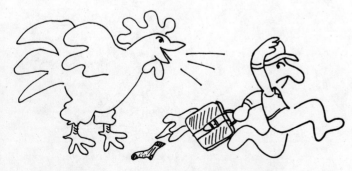

The crowing cock puts demons to flight.

Am I so cock-sure that I overlook the need for strength and balance?

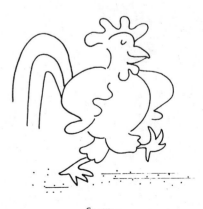

Strutting . . .

kukkutasana

COCK

Does pride lock me into position?

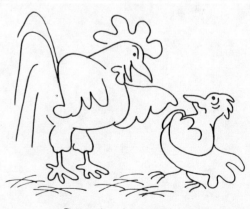

The cock is domineering.

kukkutasana

COCK

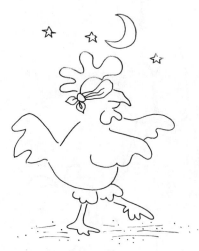

As the cock is blind at night,
the earnest aspirant also should be blind
to the temptation of the senses.

kukkutasana

COCK

mayurasana

PEACOCK

Mayura means "peacock." In this pose, the hands are placed on the floor facing backward with the little fingers touching. The body is lifted up parallel to the floor, the upper arms supporting the chest.

Pincha Mayurasana is the peacock feather pose. The forearms and hands are placed firmly on the floor, the head raised. The legs are lifted up so that torso and legs are perpendicular to the floor. The pose resembles a peacock feather or a peacock with its tail raised.

MY REFLECTIONS ON PEACOCK:

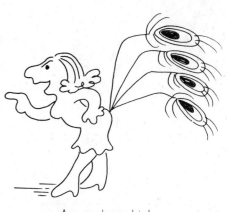

A quarrelsome bird

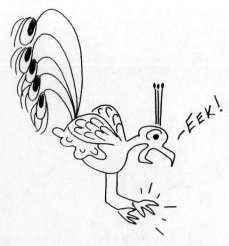

It is said that when the peacock
sees its feet, it screams, realizing how
ugly they are in contrast to its beautiful plumage.

mayurasana

PEACOCK

Does pride blind me to my ugly side?

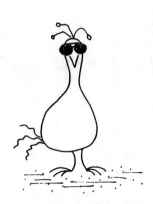

The peacock hides itself when it loses
its tail feathers and becomes ugly.

mayurasana

PEACOCK

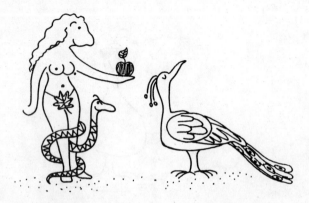

The peacock was the only bird that did not eat
of the forbidden fruit in the garden of Eden.

mayurasana

PEACOCK

Can beauty be a symbol of my aspirations, of perfection beyond the wordly kind?

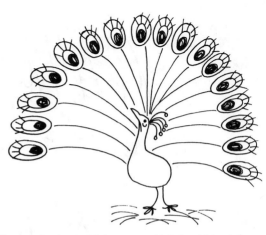

The hundred eyes of the peacock's tail point to vigilance.

mayurasana

PEACOCK

garudasana

EAGLE

Garuda is the eagle, the king of birds and the vehicle of Vishnu. This pose requires great concentration and balance as the weight is entirely on one leg with the thigh of the other leg in front, the lower leg behind, and the toes around the inner side of the ankle of the standing leg. The upper arms are held forward and parallel to the floor, with the forearms twisted around each other so that the palms of the hands are together. The pose is repeated standing on the other leg, the arms reversed.

MY REFLECTIONS ON EAGLE:

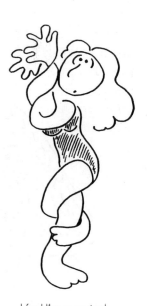

I feel like a pretzel —
trapped, wound up . . .

garudasana

EAGLE

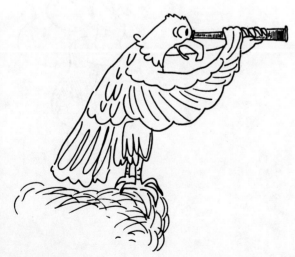

Spotting trouble from a distance in time to take action

garudasana

EAGLE

Can I see through my traps?

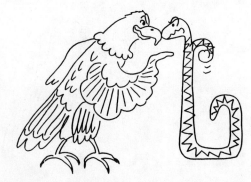

In all of us, the conflict between the eagle, the spiritual,
and the snake, temptation, is the ongoing struggle.

garudasana

EAGLE

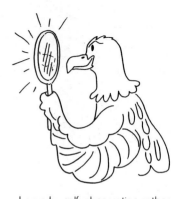

Learn by self-observation rather
than by trial and error.

garudasana

EAGLE

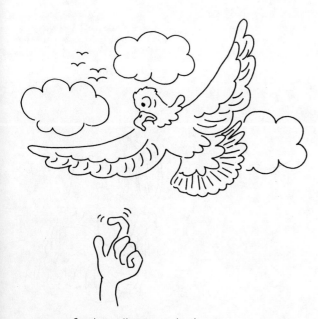

Can I soar like an eagle above
the temptations of life?

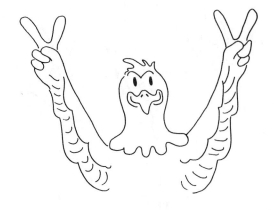

The eagle is a symbol of victory:
What are my victories?

garudasana

EAGLE

bakasana

CRANE

Baka means "crane." In this pose, the hands and arms support the weight of the body. The legs are bent, the shins resting on the backs of the upper arms, the feet together below the buttocks and off the ground.

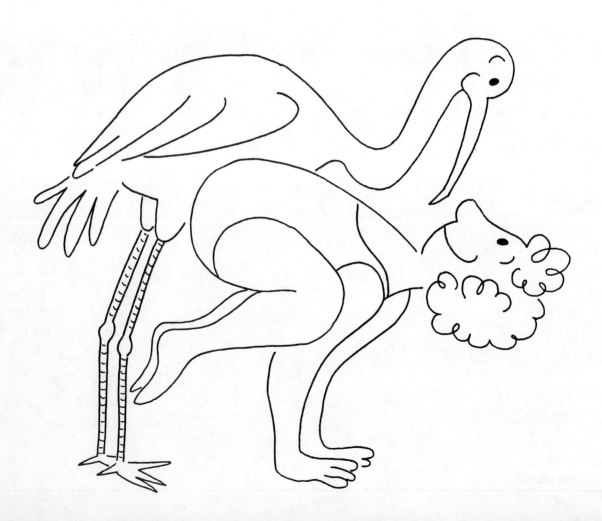

MY REFLECTIONS ON CRANE:

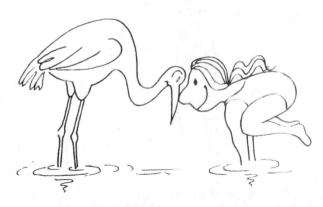

In this pose, the body resembles that of a crane wading in a pool of water.

bakasana

CRANE

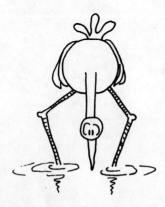

What is the water I am standing in:
the imagination? the emotions? the unconscious?

bakasana

CRANE

Do I have enough strength to reach the point of balance and vigilance? Can I find that point in my life?

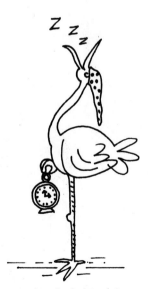

The crane has the habit of sleeping while standing on one leg.

bakasana

CRANE

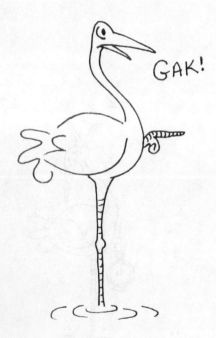

GAK!

In India the crane, by its cry,
makes known to other forms
of life the good fortune or
disaster that is about to befall them.

bakasana
CRANE

What are my distractions? What am I afraid of?

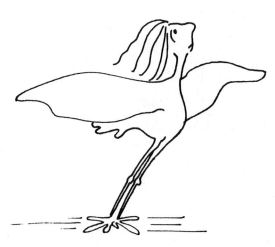

The desire to take flight, and the difficulties of spreading one's wings . . . .

bakasana

CRANE

hamsasana

SWAN

Hamsa means "swan."
In this pose, the palms
are on the floor with
the thumbs touching,
the hands facing
forward. With elbows
bent and supporting
the diaphragm, the
body is lifted up
parallel to the floor.

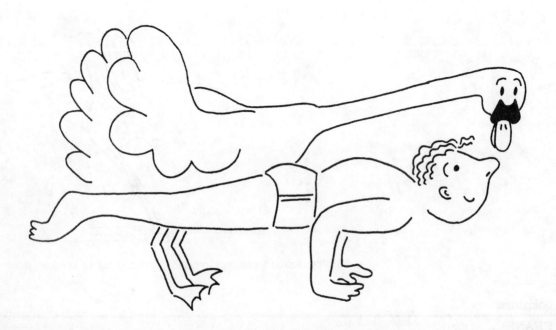

MY REFLECTIONS ON SWAN:

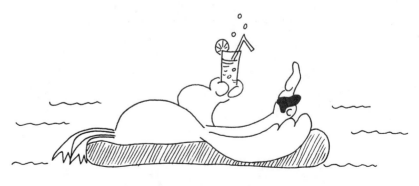

Swans are found only in calm waters.

hamsasana

SWAN

Do I allow majestic thoughts to come in — beautiful thoughts as pure as a swan?

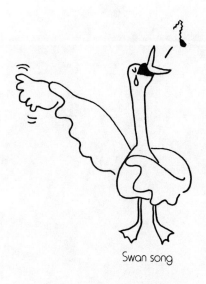

Swan song

hamsasana

SWAN

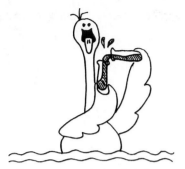

The swan is symbolic of wisdom:
it can separate milk from water
when they are mixed.

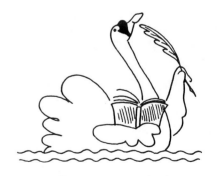

The swan enjoys solitude
and retreat being called the
"bird of the poet."

hamsasana

SWAN

Can you bring together the one swan — your physical earthly nature — with the other — your intangible spiritual nature?

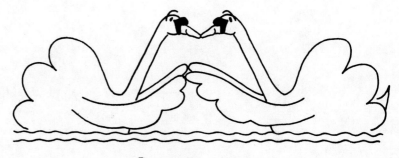

The two selves in harmony

hamsasana

SWAN

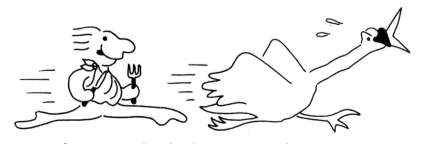

Deuteronomy admonishes that swans must not be eaten.

hamsasana

SWAN

ANIMALS

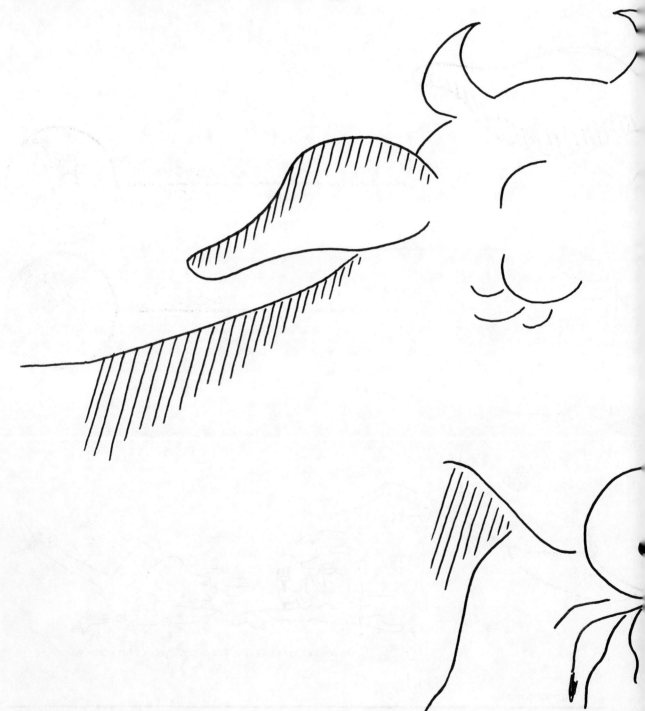

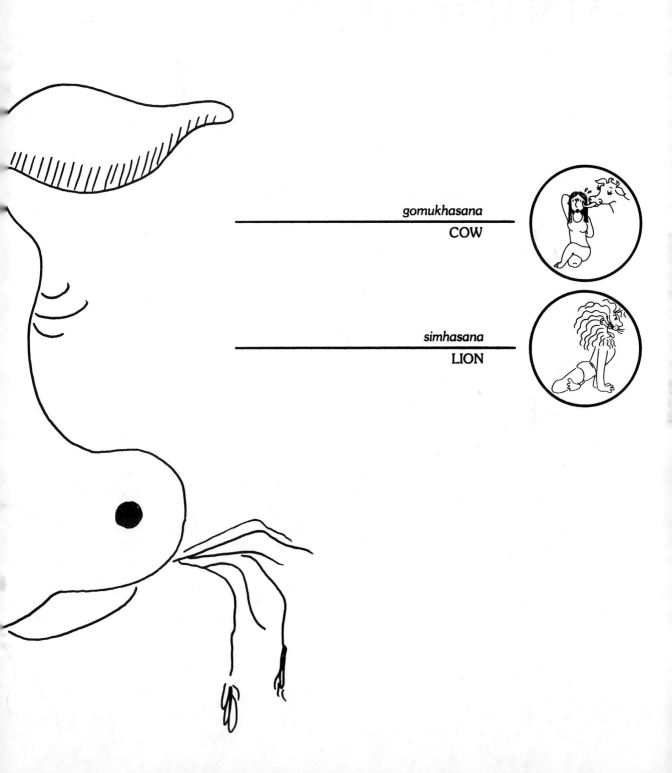

gomukhasana
COW

simhasana
LION

gomukhasana
COW-FACE

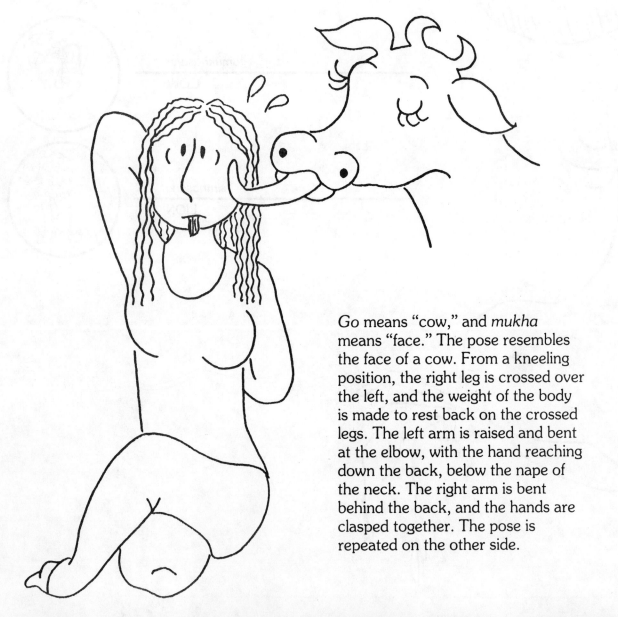

Go means "cow," and *mukha* means "face." The pose resembles the face of a cow. From a kneeling position, the right leg is crossed over the left, and the weight of the body is made to rest back on the crossed legs. The left arm is raised and bent at the elbow, with the hand reaching down the back, below the nape of the neck. The right arm is bent behind the back, and the hands are clasped together. The pose is repeated on the other side.

MY REFLECTIONS ON COW-FACE:

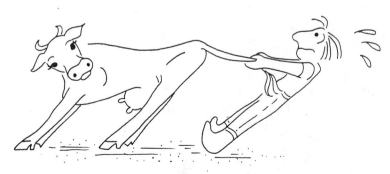

The Indian saint, Ramakrishna, compared aspirants to cows:
some you have to get by the tail backward into the temple,
while others will find their way by themselves.

gomukhasana

COW-FACE

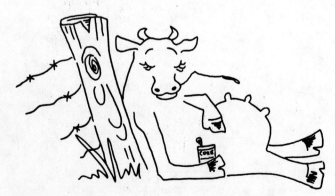

I wish I could just lie in a field like a contented cow, chewing my cud.

gomukhasana

COW-FACE

What restricts me, making me feel like a stupid cow?

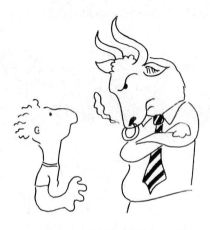

Bull-headed

gomukhasana

COW-FACE

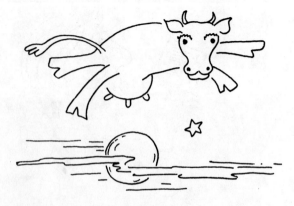

Jumping over the moon

What is the milk of Divine Wisdom that nourishes me on the spiritual path?

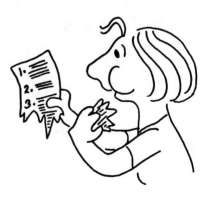

The aspirant must "chew over" spiritual
instructions to be able to digest them.

gomukhasana

COW-FACE

simhasana

LION

Simha means "lion": this pose resembles a lion roaring. The right foot is under the left buttock, and the left foot is under the right buttock. The weight is forward on the knees, and the arms are straight with the palms of the hands on the knees. (A variation is to sit in Padmasana with the weight forward on the hands which are on the floor.) The jaws are wide open, and the tongue stretched out toward the chin. The breath is forcefully exhaled with the throat open.

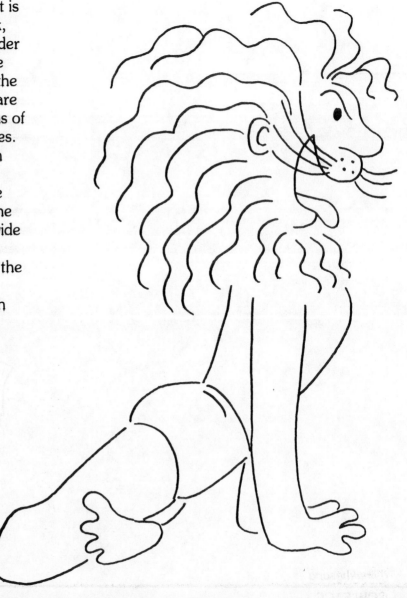

MY REFLECTIONS ON LION:

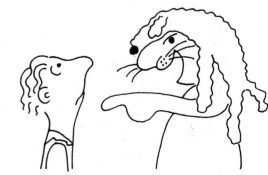

Is my power camouflaged — am I pretending to be a lamb?

simhasana

LION

Am I choking back words or tears that need to be expressed?

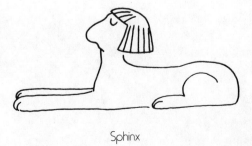

Sphinx

simhasana

LION

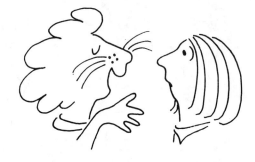
Being catty

In order to regain their strength, lions take a lot of time to rest.

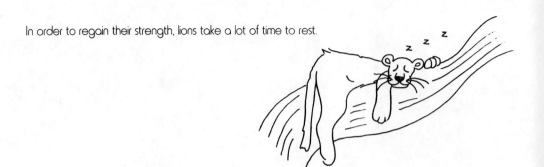

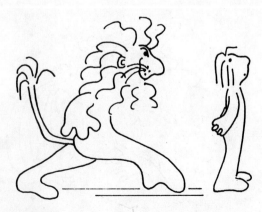

A lion will never attack straight on, but will come from the back.

simhasana

LION

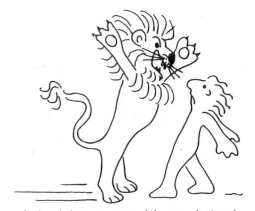

In the darkest moments of life, it can feel as if
you were being thrown into the lion's den, to be devoured.

simhasana

LION

MY REFLECTIONS ON OTHER ANIMALS:

additional

ANIMALS

SHAVASANA

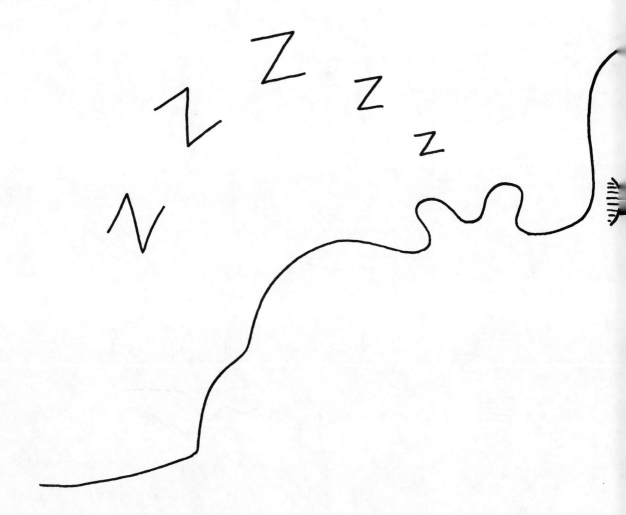

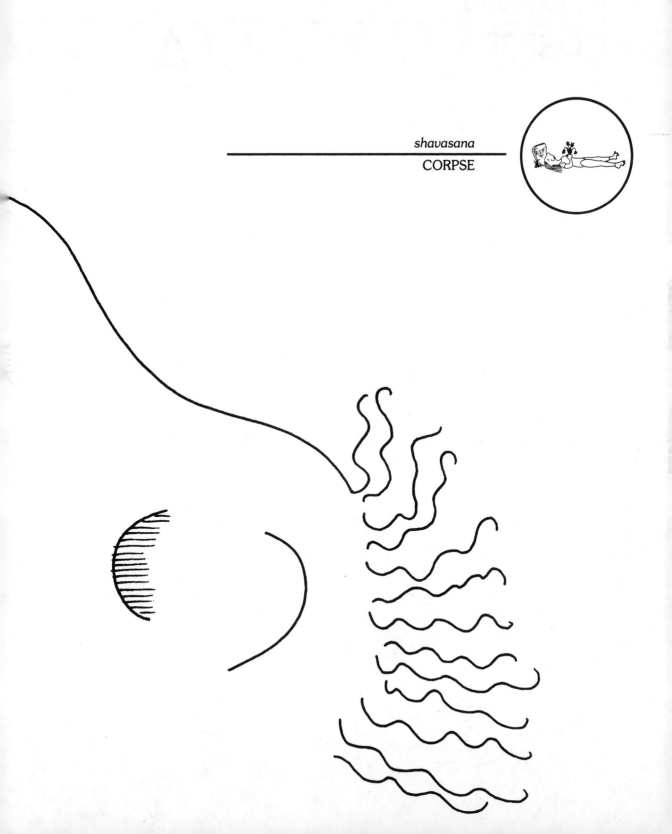

shavasana

CORPSE

shavasana

CORPSE

Shava means "corpse." In this pose, the body lies on the floor face-up and completely relaxed, while the mind is alert. The eyes are closed, the arms at the sides with the palms up. The body remains as motionless as a corpse.

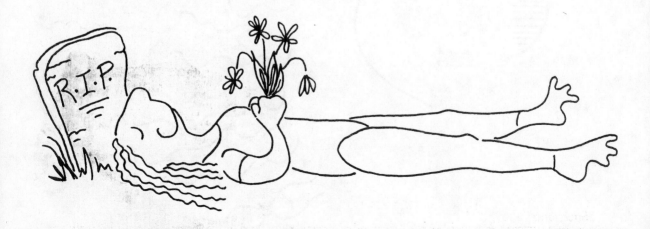

MY REFLECTIONS ON CORPSE:

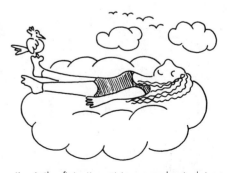

Relaxation is the first attempt to surrender, to let go.

shavasana

CORPSE

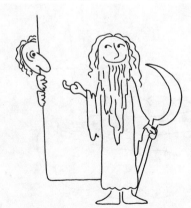

Life and death have to meet.

Is death the end of all?

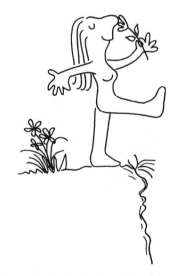

We are fearful of death, and yet we
toy with life and death as if they
were not our concern.

shavasana

CORPSE

Of all life experiences that have taken place, which were accepted by the mind? Which rejected or misconstrued?

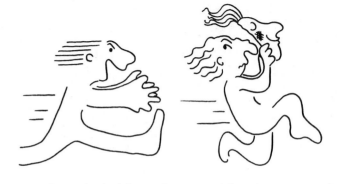

Put to death all the interfering personality aspects
that masquerade, deceive, and mislead.

shavasana

CORPSE

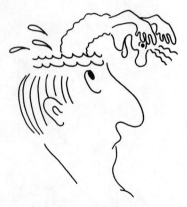

Threatening thoughts roam the
murky waters of the mind.

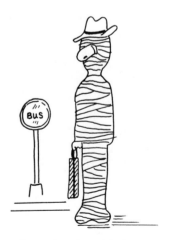

If you do not want to be a
living corpse, then the purpose
of life has to be established.

shavasana

CORPSE

ADDITIONAL REFLECTIONS:

additional
REFLECTIONS

additional

REFLECTIONS